LOW RESIDUE DIET COOKBOOK

A complete beginner guide to cure IBs, diverticulitis, and loss weight

Glen N. Quirk

Copyright © 2023 by [Glen N. Quirk]

All rights reserved. No part of this publication may be reproduced, distributed, or transmitted in any form or by any means, including photocopying, recording, or other electronic or mechanical methods, without the prior written permission of the publisher, except in the case of brief quotations embodied in critical reviews and certain other noncommercial uses permitted by copyright law.

Table of content

Snacks 48

Meal plan 56

Introduction

Mary's life took an unexpected turn when she was diagnosed with diverticulitis. The excruciating pain and discomfort became a daily ordeal. Determined to regain control, Mary researched and discovered the potential benefits of a low residue diet. With cautious optimism, she embarked on this new dietary journey.

Her meals transformed into a symphony of soft textures and gentle flavors. Creamy rice porridge, tender chicken, and steamed vegetables replaced their rougher counterparts. Mary embraced nutrient-rich options like mashed bananas and easily digestible proteins. Gradually, her symptoms subsided.

Weeks turned into months, and Mary's perseverance paid off. Her body responded positively to the low residue diet, allowing her digestive system to heal. The pain became a distant memory, replaced by renewed energy and vitality. Mary's journey highlighted the power of personalized nutrition.

Empowered by her experience, she shared her story, offering hope to others seeking relief from the clutches of diverticulitis.

About the Low Residue Diet:

The low residue diet is a therapeutic eating plan designed to minimize strain on the digestive system by limiting the intake of foods high in dietary fiber. It is commonly recommended for individuals with various gastrointestinal conditions such as diverticulitis, Crohn's disease, ulcerative colitis, and irritable bowel syndrome (IBS).

The primary goal of the diet is to reduce the bulk and frequency of bowel movements, allowing inflamed or sensitive gastrointestinal tissues to heal.

Benefits and Indications:

The low residue diet offers several benefits, including decreased bowel irritation, reduced abdominal discomfort, and alleviation of symptoms associated with certain digestive disorders. It can help manage conditions characterized by inflammation, such as diverticulitis, by minimizing the need for the intestines to work vigorously. Additionally, this diet may aid in preventing complications like bowel obstructions or bleeding. It's crucial to note that the low residue diet is typically recommended as a short-term solution during flare-ups or periods of digestive distress.

Tips for Successful Implementation:

Consult a healthcare professional: Before starting the low residue diet, consult a doctor or registered dietitian to ensure it's appropriate for your specific condition and needs.

Gradual transition: Ease into the diet by gradually reducing high fiber foods over a few days to prevent sudden dietary changes that might upset your digestive system.

Focus on low fiber options: Choose refined grains, cooked fruits and vegetables, lean proteins, and dairy products to minimize fiber intake.

Stay hydrated: Drink plenty of water to maintain hydration and aid digestion.

Monitor symptoms: Keep track of how your body responds to the diet, and adjust as needed based on symptom improvements or changes.

Reintroduce fiber gradually: After symptoms subside, work with a healthcare professional to reintroduce fiber-rich foods slowly and monitor their impact.

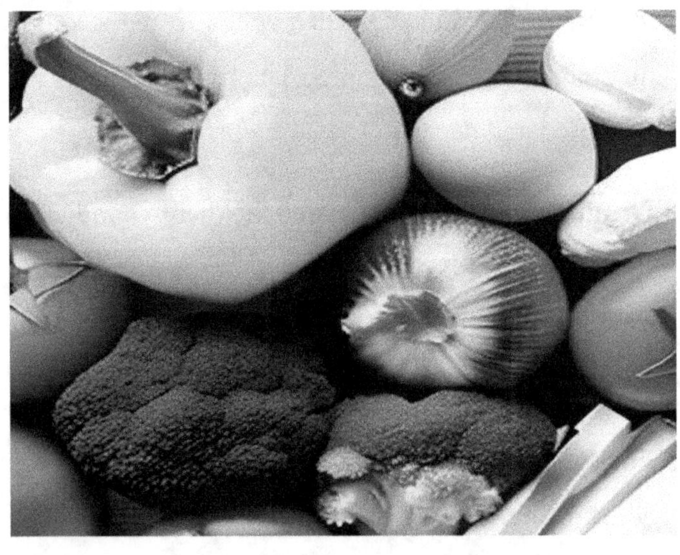

Understanding Low Residue Diet

What is a Low Residue Diet?

A low residue diet is a specialized eating plan designed to reduce the amount of undigested material passing through the gastrointestinal tract. It limits the intake of high fiber foods that can contribute to bulkier stool and increased bowel movements. This dietary approach aims to provide relief to individuals with sensitive or inflamed digestive systems, allowing their intestines to heal and recuperate.

How Fiber Affects Digestion

Fiber is an essential component of a healthy diet, as it aids digestion, promotes regular bowel movements, and supports gut health. However, for certain gastrointestinal conditions, excessive fiber intake can lead to increased bowel irritation and discomfort. Insoluble fiber, found in foods like whole grains and raw vegetables, can be particularly abrasive to inflamed or sensitive digestive tissues. By reducing fiber consumption, the digestive system's workload is lessened, providing relief and space for healing.

Conditions Requiring a Low Residue Diet

The low residue diet is often prescribed for individuals with conditions such as diverticulitis, Crohn's disease, ulcerative colitis, and irritable bowel syndrome (IBS). Diverticulitis, marked by inflamed pouches in the colon, can be exacerbated by high fiber foods. Similarly, individuals with inflammatory bowel diseases like Crohn's and ulcerative colitis may benefit from a low residue diet during flare-ups, as it can ease symptoms like abdominal pain and diarrhea. Additionally, those with IBS may find relief from bloating and cramping by temporarily adopting this diet.

In essence, a low residue diet provides a gentler approach to nutrition for those with specific digestive sensitivities, offering a chance for the gastrointestinal tract to rest and recover. However, it's important to note that the diet should only be undertaken under medical supervision and for

limited periods, as it may lack certain nutrients if
followed in the long term.

Recipe

Breakfast

Creamy Rice Porridge

Ingredients:

1/2 cup white rice

2 cups water or low-fat milk

Pinch of salt

Preparation:

Rinse the rice thoroughly.

In a pot, combine rice, water or milk, and salt.

Cook on low heat, stirring occasionally, until the rice is soft and creamy (about 20-25 minutes).

Instructions:

Serve warm. Optional toppings: mashed banana, cinnamon, or a drizzle of honey.

Serving Size: 1 cup

Nutrition (approximate):

Calories: 200

Carbohydrates: 45g

Protein: 4g

Fat: 0.5g

Fiber: 0g

Soft Scrambled Eggs

Ingredients:

2 eggs

2 tablespoons low-fat milk

Salt and pepper to taste

Preparation:

Mix the milk, eggs, salt, and pepper in a bowl.

Heat a non-stick skillet over low heat.

Pour egg mixture into the skillet and gently scramble until cooked.

Instructions:

Serve with soft white bread or well-cooked rice.

Serving Size: 2 eggs

Nutrition (approximate):

Calories: 180

Carbohydrates: 2g

Protein: 14g

Fat: 12g

Fiber: 0g

(Note: Depending on the exact components and portion amounts, nutritional values may differ.)

Banana Oat Pancakes

Ingredients:

1 ripe banana, mashed

1/2 cup quick oats

1 egg

1/2 teaspoon vanilla extract

Preparation:

In a bowl, combine mashed banana, oats, egg, and vanilla extract.

Mix until well combined.

Instructions:

Cook spoonfuls of batter on a non-stick skillet until golden brown on both sides.

Serving Size: 2 pancakes

Nutrition (approximate):

Calories: 250

Carbohydrates: 45g

Protein: 7g

Fat: 6g

Fiber: 6g

(Note: Depending on the components and portion quantities, nutritional numbers are approximations only.)

Applesauce Oatmeal

Ingredients:

1/2 cup quick oats

1 cup water or low-fat milk

1/2 cup unsweetened applesauce

Cinnamon to taste

Preparation:

Combine oats and water or milk in a pot.

Cook over low heat until oats are soft and cooked.

Stir in applesauce and cinnamon.

Instructions:

Serve warm with a drizzle of honey, if desired.

Serving Size: 1 cup

Nutrition (approximate):

Calories: 220

Carbohydrates: 45g

Protein: 6g

Fat: 2g

Fiber: 6g

(Note: Depending on the exact components and portion amounts, nutritional values may differ.)

Nut Butter on Soft Bread

Ingredients:

2 slices of soft white bread

2 tablespoons nut butter (e.g., almond or peanut butter)

Preparation:

Spread nut butter on one slice of bread.

To assemble a sandwich, place the second piece on top.

Instructions:

Serve with a side of mashed banana or applesauce.

Serving Size: 1 sandwich

Nutrition (approximate):

Calories: 300

Carbohydrates: 30g

Protein: 9g

Fat: 18g

Fiber: 3g

(Note: Depending on the exact components and portion amounts, nutritional values may differ.)

Smoothie with Soft Fruits

Ingredients:

1 ripe banana

1/2 cup ripe, peeled pear or peach

1/2 cup low-fat yogurt or lactose-free yogurt

1/2 cup water or low-fat milk

Preparation:

Combine all ingredients in a blender.

Blend until smooth and creamy.

Instructions:

Serve immediately.

Serving Size: 1 cup

Nutrition (approximate):

Calories: 200

Carbohydrates: 40g

Protein: 6g

Fat: 2g

Fiber: 5g

(Note: Depending on the exact components and portion amounts, nutritional values may differ.)

Mashed Banana Pancakes

Ingredients:

1 ripe banana, mashed

1 egg

1/4 teaspoon baking powder

Preparation:

In a bowl, mix mashed banana, egg, and baking powder until well combined.

Instructions:

Cook spoonfuls of batter on a non-stick skillet until golden brown on both sides.

Serving Size: 2 pancakes

Nutrition (approximate):

Calories: 180

Carbohydrates: 35g

Protein: 6g

Fat: 3g

Fiber: 3g

(Note: Depending on the exact components and portion amounts, nutritional values may differ.)

Lunch

Creamy Chicken and Rice Soup

Ingredients:

1 cup cooked white rice

1 boneless, skinless chicken breast

2 cups low-sodium chicken broth

1/2 cup cooked and mashed carrots

Salt and pepper to taste

Preparation:

Poach the chicken breast in the chicken broth until fully cooked. Remove the chicken and shred it.

Return the shredded chicken to the broth, add mashed carrots, and bring to a gentle simmer.

Stir in cooked rice, season with salt and pepper.

Instructions:

Serve warm, portioning into bowls. Serves 2.

Nutrition (per serving):

Calories: 220 kcal

Protein: 18g

Carbohydrates: 26g

Fiber: 2g

Fat: 4g

Tofu and Vegetable Stir-Fry

Ingredients:

1/2 cup soft tofu, cubed

1 cup steamed zucchini and carrots

2 tablespoons low-sodium soy sauce

1 teaspoon sesame oil

1/2 teaspoon grated ginger

Preparation:

Heat sesame oil in a non-stick pan.

Add tofu and ginger, sauté gently until slightly browned.

Add steamed vegetables and soy sauce, stir-fry briefly.

Instructions:

Serve over well-cooked white rice. Serves 1.

Nutrition (per serving):

Calories: 280 kcal

Protein: 12g

Carbohydrates: 25g

Fiber: 4g

Fat: 15g

Baked Fish with Mashed Potatoes

Ingredients:

1 baked fish fillet (e.g., tilapia or cod)

1/2 cup mashed potatoes (made with butter and milk)

Steamed green beans as a side

Preparation:

Prepare the fish fillet by baking with gentle seasonings.

Prepare mashed potatoes using butter and milk for a creamy texture.

Steam green beans until tender.

Instructions:

Plate the baked fish with a side of mashed potatoes and steamed green beans. Serves 1.

Nutrition (per serving):

Calories: 350 kcal

Protein: 25g

Carbohydrates: 30g

Fiber: 4g

Fat: 15g

Soft Scrambled Eggs with Toast

Ingredients:

2 scrambled eggs

2 slices of white bread, toasted

1 tablespoon butter or margarine

Preparation:

Softly scramble the eggs in a non-stick pan.

Toast the bread slices until they are easy to chew.

Spread butter or margarine on the toast.

Instructions:

Serve the scrambled eggs alongside buttered toast. Serves 1.

Nutrition (per serving):

Calories: 350 kcal

Protein: 12g

Carbohydrates: 30g

Fiber: 2g

Fat: 20g

Refined Pasta with Chicken and Spinach

Ingredients:

1 cup well-cooked refined pasta (such as white pasta)

1 cooked and shredded chicken thigh

1/2 cup cooked and softened spinach

2 tablespoons low-residue sauce (such as tomato sauce)

Preparation:

Cook the pasta according to package instructions.

Cook and shred the chicken thigh.

Gently cook the spinach until softened.

Toss the pasta, chicken, spinach, and sauce together.

Instructions:

Serve the pasta mixture in a bowl. Serves 1.

Nutrition (per serving):

Calories: 420 kcal

Protein: 20g

Carbohydrates: 40g

Fiber: 2g

Fat: 18g

Creamy Carrot and Potato Mash

Ingredients:

1 cup cooked and mashed carrots

1 cup cooked and mashed potatoes

1 tablespoon butter or margarine

Salt and pepper to taste

Preparation:

Steam and mash the carrots and potatoes.

Mix in butter or margarine, salt, and pepper for flavor.

Instructions:

Serve the carrot and potato mash as a side dish.
Serves 2.

Nutrition (per serving):

Calories: 180 kcal

Protein: 2g

Carbohydrates: 30g

Fiber: 4g

Fat: 7g

Turkey and Avocado Wrap

Ingredients:

1 soft flour tortilla

2 slices of deli turkey

1/4 avocado, sliced

Lettuce and tomato slices

Preparation:

Lay out the tortilla and layer with turkey, avocado, lettuce, and tomato.

Roll up the tortilla tightly.

Instructions:

Serve the wrap with a side of mashed potatoes or yogurt. Serves 1.

Nutrition (per serving):

Calories: 350 kcal

Protein: 18g

Carbohydrates: 30g

Fiber: 6g

Fat: 15g

Chicken and Rice Congee

Ingredients:

1/2 cup cooked white rice

1 cooked and shredded chicken breast

4 cups low-sodium chicken broth

Chopped green onions for garnish

Preparation:

Simmer the chicken broth and cooked rice in a pot.

Add the shredded chicken and let it cook gently.

Serve garnished with chopped green onions.

Instructions:

Ladle the congee into bowls. Serves 2.

Nutrition (per serving):

Calories: 280 kcal

Protein: 20g

Carbohydrates: 30g

Fiber: 1g

Fat: 7g

Tofu and Vegetable Stir-Fry

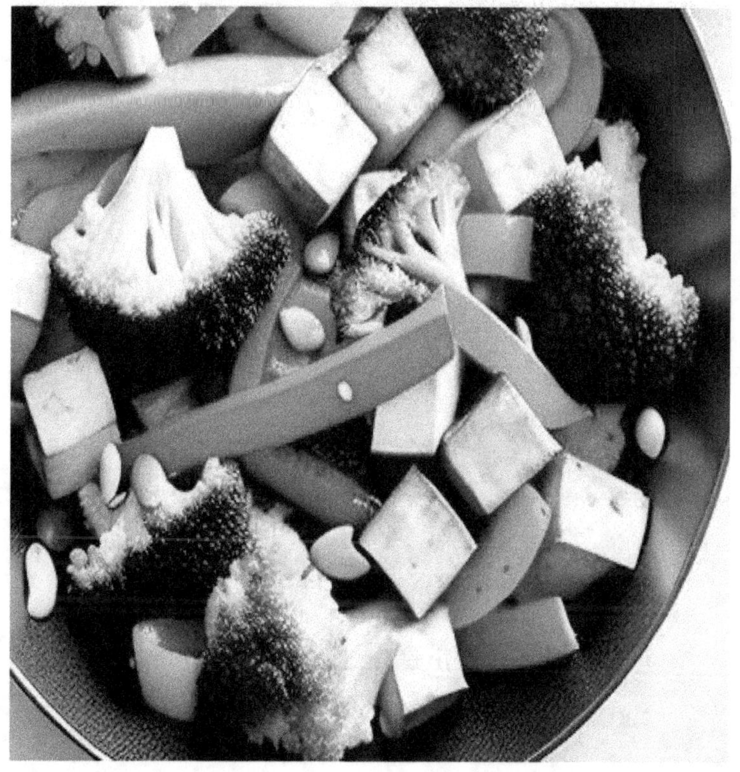

Dinner

Baked Lemon Herb Chicken

Ingredients:

4 boneless, skinless chicken breasts

2 tablespoons olive oil

1 lemon (juice and zest)

1 teaspoon dried herbs (thyme, rosemary, oregano)

Preparation:

Preheat oven to 375°F (190°C).

Place chicken breasts in a baking dish.

In a bowl, mix olive oil, lemon juice, lemon zest, and dried herbs.

Pour the mixture over the chicken.

Bake for 25-30 minutes or until the chicken is cooked through.

Instructions: Serve with steamed carrots and mashed potatoes.

Serving Size: 1 chicken breast with sides.

Nutrition Value (approx.): Calories: 300, Protein: 30g, Carbohydrates: 10g, Fat: 15g, Fiber: 2g.

Grilled Salmon with Quinoa

Ingredients:

4 salmon fillets

1 cup quinoa

2 cups low sodium chicken broth

Salt and pepper to taste

Preparation:

Rinse quinoa under cold water.

In a pot, bring chicken broth to a boil, then add quinoa.

Simmer for 15 to 20 minutes on low heat with the lid on.

Season salmon fillets with salt and pepper.

Grill salmon for 4-5 minutes per side.

Instructions: Serve grilled salmon over cooked quinoa.

Serving Size: 1 salmon fillet with quinoa.

Nutrition Value (approx.): Calories: 350, Protein: 30g, Carbohydrates: 30g, Fat: 12g, Fiber: 4g.

Turkey and Rice Stuffed Bell Peppers

Ingredients:

4 bell peppers

1 cup cooked ground turkey

1 cup cooked white rice

1 cup tomato sauce

Salt, pepper, and herbs to taste

Preparation:

Preheat oven to 350°F (175°C).

Cut the tops off bell peppers and remove seeds.

In a bowl, mix ground turkey, cooked rice, and seasoning.

Stuff peppers with the mixture.

Place stuffed peppers in a baking dish, pour tomato sauce over them.

Bake for 25-30 minutes.

Instructions: Serve alongside green beans that have been cooked.

Serving Size: 1 stuffed pepper.

Nutrition Value (approx.): Calories: 280, Protein: 20g, Carbohydrates: 30g, Fat: 8g, Fiber: 4g.

Poached Cod with Mashed Cauliflower

Ingredients:

4 cod fillets

1 head cauliflower

1 tablespoon butter

Salt and herbs to taste

Preparation:

Steam or boil cauliflower until soft.

Mash cauliflower with butter and seasoning.

Season cod fillets with salt and herbs.

Poach cod in simmering water for 6-8 minutes.

Instructions: Serve poached cod over mashed cauliflower.

Serving Size: 1 cod fillet with mashed cauliflower.

Nutrition Value (approx.): Calories: 250, Protein: 30g, Carbohydrates: 15g, Fat: 8g, Fiber: 5g.

Tofu and Vegetable Stir-Fry

Ingredients:

1 block of firm tofu, cubed

Assorted low fiber vegetables (zucchini, carrots, bell peppers)

Low sodium stir-fry sauce

1 tablespoon sesame oil

Preparation:

Press tofu to remove excess moisture, then cube.

Add tofu to a skillet of heated sesame oil.

Stir-fry until tofu is golden, then set aside.

Stir-fry vegetables until tender.

Add tofu back to the pan, pour stir-fry sauce, and cook briefly.

Instructions: Serve over well-cooked white rice.

Serving Size: 1 cup of tofu and vegetable stir-fry with rice.

Nutrition Value (approx.): Calories: 320, Protein: 15g, Carbohydrates: 40g, Fat: 12g, Fiber: 4g.

Creamy Spinach and Chicken Pasta

Ingredients:

2 boneless, skinless chicken breasts

2 cups cooked pasta

2 cups baby spinach

1 cup low sodium chicken broth

1/4 cup heavy cream

Preparation:

Season chicken with salt and pepper, then grill or sauté until cooked.

Cook pasta according to package instructions.

In a separate pan, heat chicken broth and heavy cream.

Add spinach and let it wilt.

Stir in cooked pasta and sliced chicken.

Instructions: Serve creamy pasta with a side salad.

Serving Size: 1 cup of pasta with chicken and spinach.

Nutrition Value (approx.): Calories: 400, Protein: 25g, Carbohydrates: 40g, Fat: 15g, Fiber: 2g.

Roasted Root Vegetables with Herbs

Ingredients:

Assorted root vegetables (carrots, parsnips, potatoes)

2 tablespoons olive oil

Fresh or dried herbs (rosemary, thyme)

Preparation:

Peel and chop root vegetables into bite-sized pieces.

Toss with olive oil and herbs.

Spread on a baking sheet and roast at 400°F (200°C) for 25-30 minutes.

Instructions: Serve as a side dish with grilled chicken.

Serving Size: 1 cup of roasted root vegetables.

Nutrition Value (approx.): Calories: 180, Protein: 3g, Carbohydrates: 30g, Fat: 7g, Fiber: 4g.

Eggplant and Tomato Casserole

Ingredients:

1 large eggplant, sliced

2 cups low sodium tomato sauce

1 cup shredded mozzarella cheese

Olive oil, salt, and herbs

Preparation:

Preheat oven to 375°F (190°C).

Brush eggplant slices with olive oil, sprinkle with salt and herbs.

Grill or sauté eggplant until tender.

Eggplant, tomato sauce, and cheese should be arranged in a baking dish.

Repeat layers and bake for 20-25 minutes.

Instructions: Serve with a side of cooked white rice.

Serving Size: 1 cup of eggplant and tomato casserole.

Nutrition Value (approx.): Calories: 250, Protein: 10g, Carbohydrates: 25g, Fat: 12g, Fiber: 6g.

Creamy Hummus Dip

Ingredients:

1 can (15 oz) washed and drained chickpeas

1/4 cup tahini

2 cloves garlic, minced

2 tablespoons lemon juice

2 tablespoons olive oil

Salt and pepper to taste

Preparation:

Blend the chickpeas, tahini, garlic, lemon juice, and olive oil until they are thoroughly combined.

Season with salt and pepper to taste.

Transfer to a serving bowl.

Instructions:

Serve with carrot sticks, cucumber slices, or whole wheat pita triangles.

Serving Size: 2 tablespoons

Nutrition Value: Approx. 70 calories, 3g protein, 4g fat, 6g carbohydrates

Greek Yogurt Parfait

Ingredients:

1/2 cup Greek yogurt

1/4 cup granola

1/4 cup mixed berries (blueberries, strawberries, raspberries)

Preparation:

Blended berries, granola, and Greek yogurt should be arranged in a glass or bowl.

Instructions:

Enjoy as a refreshing and protein-rich snack.

Serving Size: 1 parfait

Nutrition Value: Approx. 180 calories, 12g protein, 5g fat, 24g carbohydrates

Rice Cake with Nut Butter

Ingredients:

2 rice cakes

2 tablespoons almond butter or peanut butter

Sliced banana

Preparation:

Each rice cake should have nut butter applied uniformly.

Top with sliced banana.

Instructions:

A satisfying blend of textures and flavors.

Serving Size: 2 rice cakes

Nutrition Value: Approx. 230 calories, 6g protein, 12g fat, 27g carbohydrates

Cottage Cheese and Fruit Bowl

Ingredients:

1/2 cup low-fat cottage cheese

1/2 cup mixed fruit (melon, pineapple, grapes)

Preparation:

In a bowl, combine cottage cheese and mixed fruit.

Instructions:

A snack that is high in protein and mildly sweet.

Serving Size: 1 bowl

Nutrition Value: Approx. 120 calories, 14g protein, 1g fat, 15g carbohydrates

Veggie Sticks with Guacamole

Ingredients:

Assorted vegetable sticks (carrots, celery, bell peppers)

1 ripe avocado

1/4 onion, finely chopped

1 small tomato, diced

1 tablespoon lime juice

Salt and pepper to taste

Preparation:

Mash avocado and mix in chopped onion, diced tomato, lime juice, salt, and pepper.

Instructions:

Dip crunchy veggies into creamy guacamole.

Serving Size: 1/2 cup guacamole, with veggies

Nutrition Value: Approx. 160 calories, 2g protein, 13g fat, 11g carbohydrates

Baked Sweet Potato Fries

Ingredients:

1 medium sweet potato, cut into fries

1 tablespoon olive oil

Salt and paprika to taste

Preparation:

Preheat oven to 425°F (220°C).

Toss sweet potato fries with olive oil, salt, and paprika.

Spread on a baking sheet and bake for 20-25 minutes, flipping halfway through.

Instructions:

A healthier alternative to traditional fries.

Serving Size: 1 medium sweet potato

Nutrition Value: Approx. 140 calories, 2g protein, 4g fat, 25g carbohydrates

Apple Slices with Almond Butter

Ingredients:

1 apple, sliced

2 tablespoons almond butter

Preparation:

Spread almond butter on apple slices.

Instructions:

A crisp and satisfying combination of flavors.

Serving Size: 1 apple, with almond butter

Nutrition Value: Approx. 230 calories, 4g protein, 15g fat, 20g carbohydrates

Trail Mix

Ingredients:

1/4 cup mixed nuts (almonds, walnuts, cashews)

1/4 cup dried fruit (raisins, cranberries)

2 tablespoons dark chocolate chips

Preparation:

Mix nuts, dried fruit, and dark chocolate chips in a bowl.

Instructions:

A portable snack bursting with energy and flavor.

Serving Size: 1/2 cup

Nutrition Value: Approx. 220 calories, 5g protein, 14g fat, 20g carbohydrates

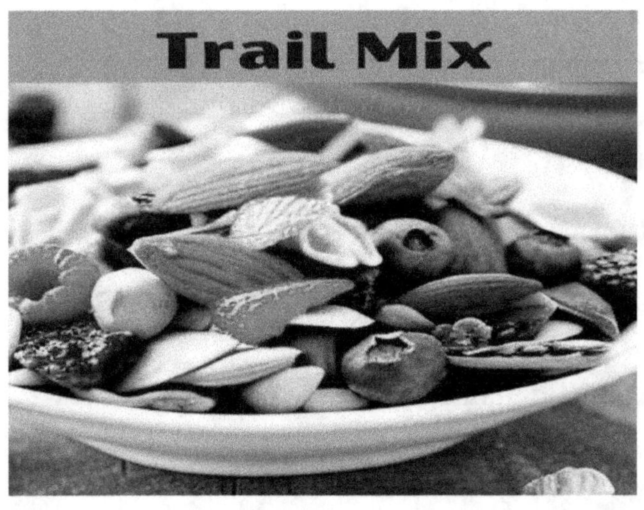

Meal plan

Day 1:

Morning: Creamy Rice Porridge

Afternoon: Clear Chicken Broth with Soft Noodles

Evening: Poached Fish with Steamed Zucchini

Day 2:

Morning: Scrambled Eggs with Soft Toast

Afternoon: Creamy Carrot Soup

Evening: Tofu Stir-Fry with White Rice

Day 3:

Morning: Banana Oat Pancakes

Afternoon: Mild Lentil Stew

Evening: Mashed Potatoes with Baked Chicken

Day 4:

Morning: Smoothie with Nut Butter

Afternoon: Clear Vegetable Broth

Evening: Quinoa with Roasted Vegetables

Day 5:

Morning: Applesauce Oatmeal

Afternoon: Creamed Spinach

Evening: Turkey Meatloaf with Gravy

Day 6:

Morning: Rice Cakes with Cottage Cheese

Afternoon: Creamy Potato Leek Soup

Evening: Poached Fish with Tender Carrot Coins

Day 7:

Morning: Soft Scrambled Eggs with Spinach

Afternoon: Chicken Broth with Refined Pasta

Evening: Silken Tofu Stir-Fry with Steamed Zucchini

Day 8:

Morning: Vanilla Rice Pudding

Afternoon: Clear Fruit Juice

Evening: Beef Stew with Soft Vegetables

Day 9:

Morning: Mashed Banana Pancakes

Afternoon: Herbal Tea and Rice Cakes

Evening: Chicken and Rice Congee

Day 10:

Morning: Creamy Rice Porridge

Afternoon: Nut Butter on Soft Bread

Evening: Baked Apple with Cinnamon

Day 11:

Morning: Scrambled Tofu with Spinach

Afternoon: Smooth Fruit Compote

Evening: Tender Roast Beef with Mashed Potatoes

Day 12:

Morning: Banana Oat Pancakes

Afternoon: Steamed Zucchini with Infused Water

Evening: Soft Tofu Stir-Fry with White Rice

Day 13:

Morning: Rice Cakes with Nut Butter

Afternoon: Creamy Carrot Soup

Evening: Delicate Seafood Pasta

Day 14:

Morning: Applesauce Oatmeal

Afternoon: Clear Vegetable Broth

Evening: Creamed Spinach with Silken Tofu

Day 15:

Morning: Smoothie with Ripe Banana

Afternoon: Poached Fish with Clear Broth

Evening: Baked Chicken with Mashed Potatoes

Day 16:

Morning: Soft Scrambled Eggs with Toast

Afternoon: Herbal Tea and Rice Cakes

Evening: Turkey Meatloaf with Smooth Gravy

Day 17:

Morning: Vanilla Rice Pudding

Afternoon: Clear Fruit Juice

Evening: Quinoa with Tender Roasted Vegetables

Day 18:

Morning: Mashed Banana Pancakes

Afternoon: Nut Butter on White Bread

Evening: Chicken and Rice Congee

Day 19:

Morning: Creamy Rice Porridge

Afternoon: Steamed Zucchini with Infused Water

Evening: Silken Tofu Stir-Fry with Tender Carrot Coins

Day 20:

Morning: Scrambled Tofu with Spinach

Afternoon: Smooth Fruit Compote

Evening: Minestrone with Refined Pasta

Feel free to interchange meals and ingredients according to your preferences and dietary requirements. Additionally, consider consulting a healthcare professional or registered dietitian to tailor the meal plan to your individual needs.

Fruits

Watermelon:

Hydration Benefit: Watermelon is composed of over 90% water, making it an excellent hydrating fruit.

Portion: 1 to 2 cups of diced watermelon.

Suitable Time: Mid-morning or as a refreshing afternoon snack.

Hygiene: Wash the watermelon thoroughly before cutting. The refrigerator is the best place to keep sliced portions.

Cantaloupe:

Hydration Benefit: Cantaloupe is water-rich and packed with vitamins.

Portion: 1 to 1.5 cups of cubed cantaloupe.

Suitable Time: As a morning or mid-afternoon snack.

Hygiene: Rinse the outside before slicing. Store cut pieces covered in the fridge.

Honeydew Melon:

Hydration Benefit: Honeydew melon is hydrating and a good source of vitamins C and B.

Portion: 1 to 1.5 cups of honeydew cubes.

Suitable Time: As a light breakfast or afternoon snack.

Hygiene: Wash the exterior before cutting, and store cut portions in the refrigerator.

Oranges:

Hydration Benefit: Oranges are rich in water and provide a dose of vitamin C.

Portion: 1 medium-sized orange or 1 cup of orange segments.

Suitable Time: As a morning fruit or in-between meals.

Hygiene: Wash the peel thoroughly, peel carefully, and store in a cool, dry place.

Grapes:

Hydration Benefit: Grapes are juicy and contribute to hydration.

Portion: A small bunch (about 1 cup).

Suitable Time: Snack on grapes during mid-morning or in the afternoon.

Hygiene: Rinse grapes thoroughly under cold water before eating.

Cucumber:

Hydration Benefit: While technically a fruit, cucumbers are mostly water and very hydrating.

Portion: 1 cup of sliced cucumber.

Suitable Time: Include cucumbers in salads or enjoy them as a light side.

Hygiene: Wash the cucumber skin well before slicing. Store unused portions in the refrigerator.

Berries (Strawberries, Blueberries, Raspberries):

Hydration Benefit: Berries are high in water content and antioxidants.

Portion: About 1 cup of mixed berries.

Suitable Time: Enjoy them as part of breakfast, a snack, or dessert.

Hygiene: Wash berries gently before consumption and store in the refrigerator.

Tips

Stay Consistent: Aim to incorporate hydrating fruits regularly into your daily routine for sustained hydration benefits.

Variety Matters: Rotate between different hydrating fruits to ensure a diverse nutrient intake and prevent taste fatigue.

Combine with Water: Enjoy hydrating fruits with a glass of water to enhance their hydrating effect.

Pre-Portion for Convenience: Pre-cut fruits into appropriate portions for easy grab-and-go snacking, promoting consistent hydration throughout the day.

Watch for Signs of Ripeness: Choose fruits that are ripe, as they tend to have higher water content and better flavor.

Mind the Fiber Content: While these fruits are low residue, they still contain some fiber. Monitor how your body responds and adjust portion sizes as needed.

Natural Sweetness: Fruits like watermelon, cantaloupe, and berries offer natural sweetness without added sugars, making them ideal for satisfying cravings.

Temperature Matters: Enjoy chilled fruits for an added cooling effect, especially during hot weather.

Pair with Protein: Consider pairing hydrating fruits with a source of protein like Greek yogurt or nuts for a balanced and satisfying snack.

Portion Control: While these fruits are hydrating, consuming them in moderation alongside a well-rounded diet is key to overall health.

Choose Fresh and Local: Opt for fresh, locally sourced fruits when available for maximum flavor and nutritional value.

Practice Proper Storage: Store fruits correctly to maintain freshness and quality. Some fruits may last longer when stored in the refrigerator.

Mindful Eating: Eat slowly and mindfully, savoring the flavors and textures of hydrating fruits.

Be Hygienic: Wash fruits thoroughly under running water before consumption, even if you plan to peel them.

Conclusion

Nourishing Wellness Through Low Residue Delights

As we come to the end of this culinary journey, we hope that this cookbook has served as a valuable guide on your path to embracing a low residue diet. The recipes, insights, and tips provided within these pages are not only meant to address specific dietary needs but also to inspire a deeper connection between nourishment and well-being.

By delving into the world of low residue cooking, you've embarked on a voyage of culinary creativity and health-conscious exploration. Through careful selection of ingredients, mindful preparation techniques, and a focus on hydration-rich foods, you've paved the way for digestive comfort and overall vitality.

Remember that the low residue diet is not just a dietary adjustment; it's a way of fostering a healthier relationship with food and self-care. As you continue to incorporate these recipes into your lifestyle, adapt them to your preferences, and explore new avenues of culinary satisfaction, may you find solace in knowing that you are nurturing your body and spirit.

As you move forward, be sure to consult with healthcare professionals for personalized guidance, and remember that health and wellness are lifelong endeavors. We extend our heartfelt gratitude for choosing this cookbook as a companion on your journey toward nourishing wellness through low residue delights. May each meal bring you joy, vitality, and a renewed sense of connection with your own well-being.

www.ingramcontent.com/pod-product-compliance
Lightning Source LLC
Chambersburg PA
CBHW050852260726
48660CB00006B/2583